MW01487880

The Secrets of Penis Enlargement

The Largely Unknown Techniques Used by Porn Stars to Grow the Penis. Learn How to Increase Several Inches Permanently!

Alessandro Clark

THE SECRETS OF PENIS ENLARGEMENT

The information provided herein is stated to be truthful and consistent, in that any liability, in terms of inattention or otherwise, by any usage or abuse of any policies, processes, or directions contained within is the solitary and utter responsibility of the recipient reader. Under no circumstances will any legal responsibility or blame be held against the publisher for any reparation, damages, or monetary loss due to the information herein, either directly or indirectly.

Respective authors own all copyrights not held by the publisher.

The information herein is offered for informational purposes solely, and is universal as so. The presentation of the information is without contract or any type of guarantee assurance.

The trademarks that are used are without any consent, and the publication of the trademark is without permission or backing by the trademark owner. All trademarks and brands within this book are for clarifying purposes only and are the owned by the owners themselves, not affiliated with this document.

THE SECRETS OF PENIS ENLARGEMENT

TABLE OF CONTENTS

INTRODUCTION

How many times have you ever felt less than confident in bed, worried about what your partner might think about the size of your penis? Have you ever wished that you had a much bigger penis and wondered how it would impact your sex life?

Men from a lot of cultures feel incredibly pressured to perform well in bed and to please their partners, and for a lot, penis size is largely connected to sexual prowess.

For a lot of people, talking about penis size is taboo. Because of this, it is not a topic that is generally talked about and discussed, which results in lots of myths and misconceptions around it.

Probably the biggest mistake regarding penis size is that "you are stuck with whatever you have."

Most men know that the male enhancement and penis enlargement industries are full of charlatans, frauds, and fake products. Scam e-mails and ads are mainly to blame in this regard; pretty much every man with internet connection has got a penis enlargement pill e-mail in their inbox or seen a male enhancement ad while browsing sites with adult-oriented content.

Some believe that the only way to permanently increase the size of their penis is by undergoing dangerous surgery that might have irreversible side effects that can drastically affect their quality of life.

Mostly because of the above, most men (and women too) believe that male enhancement is a fraud or a scam. This is no surprise due to how hard it is to separate the real information from the scams and frauds.

In this guide, I have only included information that has been proven to work consistently for a large number of men. There are no upsells or other products that you need to acquire to see real results; all you need is some willpower to remain consistent with the strategies that we will talk about in further chapters.

By reading this guide, you've taken a crucial step towards changing your life.

I'm not exaggerating: for most men, increasing their penis size will bring them a host of positive effects, many of which are not exclusively physiological but psychological and emotional as well. Partners will also appreciate and welcome these changes in most instances.

But first, we need to state the obvious: there is no such thing as a magic bullet in male enhancement.

Although it would be pretty cool if we could somehow permanently grow our penises 3 inches in a couple of weeks, this is entirely unrealistic and is what most scam ads for fraudulent products use to lure in desperate customers to make the purchase.

The good news is that pretty much every male can see substantial gains in both thickness and length if they are consistent with the strategies and techniques described in the following chapters.

A lot of men might be disappointed at the fact that there is no realistic way to grow their penis 3 inches naturally in a couple of weeks. However, if this were the case, then there would be lots of men with penises that are larger than average and there would be nothing special about them. The information you will read in this book remains mostly unknown in the mainstream, and those that manage to stick with the strategies for a while will have a powerful tool at their disposal that will give them an advantage in the "sexual marketplace."

Not only you have the potential to change your penis size, but to increase your overall enjoyment out of life as well once you cut out a significant amount of stress and anxiety that comes from sex-related fears or worries.

It's crucial to remember that as with most things health-related, the results will vary from person to person. Most men that stick to the strategies mentioned in this book will be able to see results starting from 2-3 weeks or earlier in some cases.

This guide also includes a lot of solutions to the most common male sexual health issues, such as erectile dysfunction and low libido. There is little practical benefit to having a bigger penis if you are suffering from ED or have a total lack of health desire. The idea is to have a penis that is not only bigger than what you currently have but one that is also almost "invincible."

Thank you, and I hope that you enjoy the journey towards a more confident and healthier sex life!

CHAPTER 1: WHY DO MEN CARE SO MUCH ABOUT PENIS SIZE?

A lot of people believe that being obsessed with penis size is a new thing, mostly prevalent in western cultures. However, if we take a look at our history, we can see that several different cultures saw large male organs as something positive; they represented not only masculinity but power and strength too.

There is phallic imagery pretty much everywhere around the world. The adoration or admiration of phallic images dates back to thousands of years ago. But even nowadays some cultures revere the penis as something sacred. In the city of Kawasaki, Japan, there is a festival called Kanamara Matsuri which is held each spring that has the penis as the central theme of the event.

In this festival, families show up to celebrate fertility, sex and the creation of life. In Thimpu, Bhutan, the penis is primarily considered to be a symbol of fertility, and it also helps protect against evil spirits and even gossip. Their murals are famous for showing large penises and dragons.

It is true, however, that men are now more preoccupied with size than ever. Some are desperate enough to increase their penis in length or width that they take extreme measures. Feeling inadequate in this area may cause a lot of damage to one's self-esteem. Most men that feel inadequate due to their penis size have been found to have unhealthy self-esteem. This unhealthy self-esteem is not limited to the bedroom and often ends up spilling over to many other areas of their lives.

Men that are worried about the size of their penis take specific measures, such as avoiding public bathrooms out of fear of exposing their penis and being the subject of ridicule by others; some even abstain from sex altogether out of fear of being seen as inadequate if compared to others.

Why do we care so much about size?

As men, it is during our childhood years when we form most of our opinions and expectations about penis size. For instance, it is extremely common for a boy to see the penis of his father or older sibling and then believe that their penis is small in comparison (without being fully aware that age plays a part in penis size). This image tends to stick inside a boy's head and can be very hard to change. Even after a boy goes through puberty and his penis changes in size, the belief that their penis is smaller than usual sticks.

Boys that are considered to be late bloomers and thus, develop at a slower pace than others, are often ridiculed by boys with a more average growth rate; late bloomers are often teased in locker rooms and bathrooms by their peers with bigger penises. This ridicule can affect boys so profoundly that the anxiety and fear that results from it may last for years or even decades.

Then there are also boys that, at some point, read what the average male penis size is, and quickly feel disappointed after measuring their penis. What they haven't realized is that the penis size they are comparing to is usually to that of a fully grown adult. Also, most of these measurements are done while the penis is fully erect, as measuring a flaccid penis can sometimes be challenging and not very exact. Some boys might even be measuring their penises at a flaccid length, and further create additional anxiety when they find that their measurements are far below that of the average.

Also, boys and teenagers are more exposed to pornography than ever before. It is not uncommon for boys to begin watching adult videos before age 10. Male porn stars are often selected because their penis size is significantly above average, as it is one of those attributes that porn watchers typically expect. Because of this, a considerable amount of movies and videos feature well-endowed men.

Young boys (and even lots of men) aren't aware of this fact, and they might often compare their penises to what they see on the screen, often resulting in insecurity and anxiety. Also, a lot of men that upload homemade adult videos tend to have larger than average penises. It is not usual for men with average or below average penises to upload homemade videos, as often they may receive negative comments from viewers.

Because of this, boys that watch a lot of pornography might believe that pretty much everyone has a larger penis than they do.

What they think is the average male penis size might be much bigger than what it is. Their perception of reality has been heavily influenced by what they often see in adult videos.

Other factors may also affect men's perspective of what their penis is really like. For instance, men usually view their penises from above. Try doing the following experiment: while standing up, hold your hand at the same height where your penis is, and then move it towards eye level. See how much smaller your hand looks when you see if from above?

Real penis size

Whenever you look at penis measurements found in actual studies, it's crucial to remember that these (unless noted) have been done on adults and not on developing boys or teenagers.

There is little reason to measure the penis of a developing boy or teenager, as there will be lots of variabilities. Boy's testicles tend to grow while they are between ages eleven to eighteen. It is common for the testicles to start developing first and then the penis. We know that a man's penis doesn't stop fully growing until age 21.

The average penis size around the world for adult men is around three and a half inches and five inches when erect.

Thickness varies a lot more. Standard flaccid penis width can be anywhere from three to four inches, and erect girth is around four and four and a half inches.

Measuring erect penis size is thought to be far more critical than flaccid penis size. The reason for this is simple: the penis is typically only used in sexual activity while fully erect, so why measure it while flaccid?

Some men that have very average or even below average flaccid penis sizes but can get to even above average sizes when erect. The term "grower" applies to them. A "shower" on the other hand, is a man that has an impressive flaccid size, but who's penis doesn't grow that much when fully erect.

Measuring your penis will be crucial throughout your male enhancement journey, as it is one of the easiest ways to check your progress. To measure your penis correctly, you can use a regular ruler or measuring tape. If you are using a ruler, make sure that it is straight. Whichever method you choose (rule or measuring tape), be consistent, and do not switch from one to another as there can be slight differences. We mainly care about progress and how the penis changes over time.

To measure your penis when using a ruler, press it firmly into your groin and write down the length from the base to the very tip.

If using a measuring tape, measure as much length as possible from the base to the tip of the glans.

Penis width can be trickier to measure, and it is best to use a measuring tape for it. Wrap the tape around the fullest part of the penis.

How happy are men with their penis size?

A significant amount of men from lots of different cultures around the world tend to feel very unhappy or unsatisfied with the size of their penis.

There have been several studies done where men are surveyed and asked about how they currently feel about their penis size. It is normal for these studies to find that close to 50% of men aren't satisfied with their penis size. Most of these men say that they would be happier if their penis were bigger.

Interestingly, men with average-sized penises tend to suffer more from anxiety and insecurity than men with smaller than average penises.

Does race affect penis size?

There are lots of myths surrounding race and penis size, but there is no denying the fact that race does play a role in average penis size. The most prevalent myths surrounding penis size and race are that Asian men tend to have penises that are much smaller than average, and that African men have much larger penises than men from other races.

There has been a lot of research done on the subject of penis size around the world. There was a large study that analyzed the differences between penis size in over 100 different nationalities.

In the end, the study did find that African countries tend to have the biggest penises in the world, but even between different African countries, there are lots of variabilities. There are some countries with a predominantly Hispanic population, such as Ecuador and Venezuela have a larger average penis size than many countries with mostly African people.

Countries with a predominantly white male population such as the United States and certain European countries such as Germany and Norway tend to be somewhere in the middle of the list, with an average penis size that is around 5 inches.

Although Asian countries do seem to be smaller than others, the difference has been greatly exaggerated. For instance, the average penis size of a Japanese male is not that far away from the average American male size.

When is a penis considered truly small?

There is no clear cut answer to this, as it depends on who you are asking. For instance, if you ask a doctor when is a penis considered to be medically small (small enough to be a candidate for a penis enlargement surgical procedure), they will tell you that at three inches erect or less. Men that are above this size aren't usually candidates for penis enlargement procedures as they can have dangerous side effects.

There is a condition called a "micropenis." It is a very rare condition, as it is estimated that only around .6% of males have it. This condition can be extremely damaging for men with it. Hormonal imbalances, while the baby is inside the mother's womb, typically cause it. When fetuses are around eight weeks old, their penises start to develop. During the twelfth week, the penis has usually finished developing, and then it starts to grow. Male sex hormones are in charge of promoting penis growth.

The growth is critical during the second trimester and beyond. Certain factors can interfere with male hormone production, and end up affecting the growth of the penis. In severe cases, the penis ends up being extremely small.

Hormone therapy can be highly effective in treating micropenis in babies. Specific forms of testosterone and growth hormone therapy can help bring a micropenis to regular size. Usually, this hormonal therapy is done during childhood and after puberty to boost the development of the penis. Adults that have micropenis don't have many options available since hormone therapy won't do much at that point.

Fortunately, micropenis is not a common condition, and even men with micropenis can gain size by following a safe male enhancement routine, like the ones we will explore in further chapters.

Besides surgery, there is also a lot of research being done with regenerative medicine. While this type of research is still in its infancy, there have already been experiments done where new tissue is grown from a patient's scrotal skin. This skin is then grafted to the penis to promote size growth.

Women's views about penis size

As you probably know by now, men are far more worried about penis size than women. A lot of men believe that only a penis that is way above average is enough to satisfy a woman. There has been a lot of research done on the level of satisfaction of women with their partner's size, and it has been found that over eighty-five percent of women are happy with their partner's size. Quite a contrast with men, since 45% percent of them believe that their size is very far away from being adequate.

Of course, this doesn't mean that women don't care at all about size, but the degree to which they care has been greatly exaggerated by men and the media. It is true that for a relatively small percentage of women, size matters more than usual, but most of them are ok with an average-sized penis.

A particular experiment done on the subject took several women and showed them many different penis dimensions through the use of 3d printed images. The dimensions of the printed penis models varied quite significantly, from four to nine inches in length. The study found that women's preferences for penis size changed depending on the type of relationship they were looking for.

For instance, if a woman was looking for a short term relationship, they seemed to prefer penises that were around 6 inches in length.

On the other hand, if they were interested in a short term relationship or one night stands, they preferred penises that were slightly longer than usual.

Reality check

After reading this chapter, you might feel a bit relieved after you realize how distorted the views and expectations of men about penis size are and how they are vastly different from what women are looking want. It can be relieving to hear that it is unnecessary to have an 8+ inch penis to please your partner, even though the adult videos you've seen have tried to convince you otherwise.

Nevertheless, this guide was written primarily to help men increase their penis size permanently, regardless of what their goals are. It is merely important to know that it is not necessary to shoot for an eight or nine-inch penis.

In reality, an eight or nine-inch penis will be more than a lot of sex partners can handle comfortably.

If you are looking to increase the size of your penis to increase your self-confidence or decrease anxiety, then knowing how to do this effectively, without side-effects, can change your life for the better. Very few men (and women) know about the information included in the following chapters. It remains mostly unknown to the mainstream eye.

CHAPTER 2: DEMYSTIFYING MALE ENHANCEMENT

A quick look at the male enhancement industry is enough to confuse the average man. There are so many products available that it can be tricky to know what works and why. Most of the products available are scams and frauds, which makes it even more challenging to get to the stuff that does work.

Many of the products related to male enhancement can be very expensive. The penis is quite a complex organ with lots of sensitive tissue, so its definitively not a good idea to be experimenting with products that might put your health at risk.

In this chapter, we will take a look at the most popular products in the male enhancement industry. A lot of these products promise to add inches to your penis and/or boost your libido, erection quality, etc. By understanding what works and what doesn't, you will have a better understanding of the male enhancement industry as a whole. You will also know what you should definitively stay away from and what will help you increase in size.

Penis enlargement pills

There is arguably no other product in the world of male enhancement that is as infamous as penis pills. The average male with internet access has seen far too many penis pills ads to count. Most sites with adult content advertise these products. These pills promise the average man incredible increases in length and girth of the penis in as little as two or three weeks. Seeing ads of pills that promise a two-inch increase in length in less than a couple of weeks isn't that uncommon.

Because of how bombarded we've become with these products, most men approach them with a great deal of skepticism.

It has even become commonplace to mock penis pill ads. After all, the products they advertise sound way too good to be true.

You may be asking yourself what exactly do penis pills (if anything) or why some men continue to buy them. After all, a lot of them offer a money-back guarantee, so what gives? You also might be wondering if they pose any health risks.

Let's cut to the chase; pills do not work at all. Here's why. These products usually contain a list of "sneaky" ingredients (such as horny goat weed and maca) that give some men the illusion that they're gaining size. What these ingredients usually do is increase the erection quality of the penis or boost libido.

While taking them, there can be an increase in circulation that improves erection quality (which means a slight temporary boost in size). Having more blood flow in the penis area means a larger and longer erection.

For men that experience these effects, they might quickly assume that the penis pills are giving them a visible increase in size. A lot of penis pills sellers offer a 30-day money-back guarantee. They know that a lot of men taking these pills will receive a temporary boost in erection quality and, as a consequence, won't be returning the pills. Some of these pills also boost the libido, so men continue to take them without complaints.

These pills usually aren't dangerous, but there is very little regulation involved in their production, so it is essential to check the list of ingredients before taking any of these supplements. They also tend to be extremely expensive, so there is little reason for someone to recommend them to improve erection quality and/or libido.

In reality, these pills do very little to increase the size of the penis permanently. Improvements in erection quality will only be temporary. Once you stop taking these pills, you will be back to where you started.

Penis enhancement surgery

A lot of men might have heard about penis enhancement surgery, and out of all the "mainstream" options it is widely regarded as being the one that most believe will give good results. There's quite some truth to this. A surgeon with proper training can potentially change the lives of a lot of men.

However, just as with most surgical procedures, there is always a possibility of complications and side effects. It can be tricky to get the results you exactly want with a penis enhancement surgery. A common side effect of this surgery is temporary erectile dysfunction, and in some cases, it can even be permanent.

Patients must take proper care of themselves after surgery to diminish the risk of any unwanted complications. While complications aren't the norm, it is crucial to be aware of the life-altering side effects that may occur.

Male enhancement surgery is beyond the scope of this guide and is a quite extense medical topic in itself. It is essential to know that it is always there but should only be used as the last resort, especially when there are much safer alternatives to try first.

A lot of men that like to have things the quick way might be tempted to try surgery, as it is an "instant" solution to their problem. However, once you add in the recovery time and the possible complications, it is better to consider other options first in most cases.

Extenders

Let's start analyzing some of the most common devices in the male enhancement world. There are lots of tools being sold that promise to add many inches to the penis. Some of these devices can even be quite practical because they can be worn while wearing clothes, and can be used in a "set and forget" fashion, so you don't have to interrupt your daily activities such as working or doing chores at home. Penis extenders fall into this category.

You might be wondering if these extender devices do work or not, and the answer might surprise you: in most cases, they do work. How they work is nothing new. A lot of cultures around the world have been experimenting with tools to apply continuous resistance to several parts of their bodies to help them increase in size. For instance, in some cultures, such as the Padaung tribe in Thailand, having a long neck is a very desirable trait for women.

To achieve this length, women add rings to their necks that apply constant pressure to the tissue, helping it expand with enough time. Women continue to add rings to their necks to achieve their desired size.

You may also have seen some people with enlarged earlobes. They achieve this by using earrings that expand the size of their earlobes slowly.

Interestingly enough, there are certain cultures where men have experimented with increasing the size of their penises in similar ways. In some cases, they attach heavy objects to their genitals to apply constant pressure that will trigger growth.

Penis extender devices work similarly. They apply resistance to the penis to promote tissue expansion. This force increases the size of the penis through adaptation.

They are one of the most popular devices in the male enhancement world because of how practical they can be in lots of cases. They are primarily used to add length to the penis, but some of them do help add a bit of girth.

There are a few drawbacks to penis extenders, the first being that they tend to be a bit uncomfortable and that it is almost impossible to wear them discreetly while wearing tight clothing. Most people with jobs wouldn't be able to wear them during work unless they are allowed to wear very loose clothing. When wearing baggy clothing, these devices can be virtually undetectable.

Penis extenders are typically worn anywhere between 40 minutes and 8 hours per day, based on the level of toleration and the time that you can wear them. Beginners that haven't subjected their penis tissue to much force start by wearing them just for a few minutes every day and then work up the time. To see results, it usually takes several months: anywhere from 6 to 8 months to see significant changes is reasonable.

A lot of penis extenders can be quite uncomfortable. Usually the cheaper ones are the most unpleasant ones to wear, and the most expensive ones tend to be the most comfortable because of higher quality materials and research behind their development. Some of the high-end devices are even designed to be worn during sleep, so they are convenient. However, those devices can cost several hundred dollars. Some of the budget options do work, but they tend to take longer to show results and, as mentioned, are the most uncomfortable to wear.

Penis extenders do work, but only for those that can remain consistent and can wear them for large chunks of time every day. If you are interested in a penis extender, you should go with a model that has solid research backing it up and that you make sure that you'll be able to wear it for at least the minimum time it requires to show results. Some of the lesser-known devices can even be a little dangerous, so its best to avoid them.

It's essential to be cautious with most things regarding male enhancement. If the drawbacks of high cost, time and discomfort are too much for you to handle, its best to take a look at other options.

Air-based pumps

There are two types of penis pumps commonly used for male enhancement: air-based pumps and water-based pumps. They both have their pros and cons, which we will go in detail.

Air-based pumps are popular in the mainstream, and even people that don't know anything at all about male enhancement have heard about them. They are typically used by men to help treat erectile dysfunction and prolong ejaculation. They can also help a man's libido by increasing blood flow in the genital area. Air-based pumps are not usually used for increasing penis size, but some men have reported some permanent size benefits.

Air-based pumps tend to be cheaper than water-based pumps, but they have a few drawbacks. When using the device, it is common for edema accumulation to occur in the penis after reaching a specific vacuum level. Edema can be a problem with the constant use of these devices and can cause discoloration, discomfort, and soreness in the penis.

If your main objective is to improve blood flow in the genital region and have better erections and stamina during sex, then air-based pumps could be a good option, but let's see why water-based might be superior.

Water-based pumps

Water-based pumps are not as widely known as air-based pumps, mainly because they haven't been in the market for as long. However, they are increasing in popularity every year because they provide excellent short and long term benefits.

A lot of devices in male enhancement offer either short term or long term benefits, but rarely both.

As the name suggests, water-based pumps use water to create a vacuum instead of air. You can use them while showering or bathing. The vacuum created by water-based pumps can be very intense and can force a lot of blood inside the penis. The amount of blood it can force is higher than that which a normal man can achieve via a regular erection. After a single correct use, it can increase the penis' size for a few hours. A lot of men use them just for this reason alone. They can also be used to treat erectile dysfunction or help improve erection quality.

After a few months of regular use, water-based pumps can give giving permanent thickness gains.

Edema can still build up when using water-based pumps, but it is much less of a problem.

Like air-based pumps, they also help improve overall male health by promoting blood flow in the genital region. Libido, stamina and erection quality tend to improve with regular use.

Probably the main two drawbacks of water-based pumps are that they are expensive, especially when compared to air-based pumps; they are also not as practical. You can only use them comfortably while showering or bathing after all.

Penis hanging

Penis hanging involves using a device that creates force by hanging a weight on a penis that will help promote tissue expansion overtime. It is one of the most ancient forms of male enhancement known. When the micro-tears heal, new cells grow, and the penis will inevitably increase in size when done correctly.

Penis hanging is mainly used to improve the length of the penis, but some men have reported girth increases too.

You might be wondering about the difference between penis extenders and penis hanging. They both work in a similar fashion, by creating micro-tears in the penis tissue; however, hanging applies a lot of force over a short period to promote these micro tears and extenders place very little force over a long period. They use tension and time in opposite ways.

One of the positives of this method is that you have complete control over the amount of tension that you use during a session. Just like weight lifters can choose precisely with how much weight they want to train a muscle, someone using penis hanging can decide how much tension to apply to the penis tissue.

However, penis hanging is a bit controversial as it is one that can be easily overdone if not practiced carefully, and undesirable effects can happen. It is best to avoid this option or only leave it until you are highly experienced with male enhancement.

Clamping

Penis clamping is another one of those methods that are best to leave to advanced male enhancement users. Clamping is used to increase the thickness of the penis. Why is it considered controversial, though?

To perform penis clamping correctly, you have to use a device to build significant pressure inside the penis and also to restrict the flow of blood. There will be some inflow of blood but in small amounts. After a while, the pressure forced inside the corpus cavernosum of the penis will force the tissue to grow through adaptation.

Complications can quickly occur if clamping is not performed safely especially vein thrombosis. Clamping applies a lot of pressure inside the penis, and just as with hanging, it can be very easy to go overboard and cause some damage.

Manual male enhancement exercises

A lot of people might find it hard to believe that it is possible to exercise the penis. After reading about the methods mentioned in this chapter, you are probably more open to the fact that the penis can indeed be forced to grow and expand beyond its normal size. Exercising works in a similar way that devices do: by applying force and tension and by restricting or increasing blood flow.

There are several advantages that exercises have over male enhancement devices. First of all, they're completely free.

Unlike an extender or a water-based pump, you don't need to spend hundreds of dollars, as you can perform male enhancement exercises without cost whenever you have privacy.

There are tiny drawbacks to manual exercises. Probably the biggest drawback is that you need to set aside some time to do them, unlike some devices such as penis extenders, which can be worn for hours without you having to do anything.

A cool thing about male enhancement exercises is that there are many different ones available. No matter what your goal is, there is probably an exercise that will help you get there. Some exercises are used for length gains, while others are mainly used for gaining more thickness. Other exercises help by promoting good blood flow in the penis and thus help increase the quality and strength of your erections. These exercises also help boost libido.

Another huge advantage of manual exercises is that you'll be able to see results quickly when you perform them consistently and correctly. Some men have reported seeing results in as soon as three to four months when performing them.

The type of male enhancement that this guide will focus on for length and girth gains are manual exercises. Exercising the penis is not that different from exercising muscles. After a while, the tissue will need to adapt to the force and tension you'll be applying to the penis. To continue making progress, you will need to switch things after a while, which is why there are routines included for beginners, intermediate, and advanced users.

Because male enhancement exercises are completely free and healthy when performed safely, you can begin performing them today if you wish. The earlier you start, the better if you want to see results as fast as possible.

In the next chapters, we will take a look at the routines that can be used to get to your desired size without facing any issues or setbacks. However, we will first take a detailed look at the specific exercises that will be used in the routines so that you start getting familiar with them.

CHAPTER 3: Effective and safe male enhancement exercises

It's now time to take a look at the most effective and safe (when performed correctly) male enhancement exercises available. These exercises have been the backbone of countless successful programs.

Exercise #1. Jelqs

Jelqs are probably the most known male enhancement exercises. Even people that are not well acquainted with male enhancement might have heard about jelqing.

Jelqing has been proven to be extremely useful, which is why it has been the backbone of many routines and programs. It is not unusual for men to gain up to 2 inches in length from routines that include lots of jelqing.

Jelqs are great because they not only help increase the length of your penis but the thickness too. They also promote better blood flow, resulting in stronger and firmer erections. Because of how often they are used in male enhancement, for many different purposes, you should get well acquainted with how to perform them correctly.

The term jelqing sounds a bit strange, and we don't know what its exact origins are. We do know that in western cultures, the word has been in rotation since at least the '70s. The word means milking because of the motion used for the exercise is very similar to the motion used milking a cow.

You can use your erection quality (firmer, more frequent erections) as a very accurate gauge of how well you're performing male enhancement exercises, including jelqing. If you notice an improvement in erection quality and libido after performing an exercise or a routine for a while, then that's a good sign, and you should continue with what you've been doing.

On the other hand, if you notice that your erection quality isn't improving or that it's even worsening, then that's a warning sign that you should either back down the force or intensity that you're using to perform the exercises or maybe decrease the frequency of the number of sessions you do each week.

Performing the jelqs.

For male enhancement exercises, your level of erection matters a lot, as certain exercises can only be performed with a specific erection level. Some exercises can even be unsafe when performed at a high erection level.

To simplify things, imagine that there are four erection levels.

-When the penis is flaccid, it doesn't count as an erection level. Little to no extra blood should be inside the penis.

-At the first erection level, the penis is slightly bigger than when flaccid, but not significantly so. We could say that it's a quarter or 25% erect.

-At the second erection level, the penis is now noticeably hard, but not enough to perform sexual intercourse. It's 50% erect.

-At the third level, the penis is just barely firm enough to be used in sexual intercourse. This would be a 75% erection level.

-At the fourth and last level, the penis is as erect as it can naturally be and can easily be used in sexual intercourse. This would be 100% erect, or in other words, a full erection.

Although jelqing is a very effective exercise for the penis, it can be easy to go overboard with it if you use a 100% erection level with it. Whenever you perform a new male enhancement exercise, you must keep in mind that the tissue in your penis is not yet used to the stress and tension you're applying. Because of this, it's best to go slow and use minimal force. For jelqing, it is recommended to use only use an erection level of 25% to 75%. If you use more than 75%, then you will be pushing a lot of blood towards the tip of your penis and can quickly overstimulate the tissue. The result will be that you will halt your progress due to overtraining.

Jelqing with an erection that's higher than 75% should only be done by advanced users with significant experience with the motion.

As mentioned before, exercising the penis is not that different from exercising other parts of the body, such as muscles. When you go to the gym for the first time, it is highly unlikely that you will use a massive set of weights to exercise as you wouldn't be able to exercise correctly and will probably injure yourself, making your progress much slower.

To perform the jelqing motions smoothly, you should use some lubricant. Any fluid that is safe for your skin will work ok. Two of the most used lubricants for jelqing are baby oil and Vaseline.

When performing jelqing, both hands are used to do repetitions one after the other. To start, lubricate both the penis shaft and both hands.

Try to get your penis to a level 2 erection. Levels 1 and 3 are also fine, but level 2 is usually the best. Don't get too obsessed about erection level when jelqing; the first three will all work. Never go above 75%.

When performing this exercise, you might notice that your erection level goes beyond level three without much effort. Because you aren't yet used to the jelqing motion, you might find it slightly stimulating. If this is the case, take a break for a few seconds or minutes until your erection goes below 75% and then continue. After a while, you will stop finding jelqing as stimulating, and you will be able to perform the motions more quickly with fewer setbacks.

With the index finger and thumb of one hand, form what's commonly known as the "Ok" sign or circle shape. The circle should be just big enough to grip the shaft of your penis slightly tight. It shouldn't be loose.

To perform one repetition, grip the base of the shaft of the penis. It should be as close to the pubic bone as you can manage. You then proceed by sliding the circle across the shaft of the penis while applying a slight amount of pressure with the grip while you do so. Imagine that you are pushing the blood through the shaft of the penis. You must stop right when you reach the glans area. It's crucial never to push all the way to the tip, as this can be too much and cause you to overtrain easily.

Some men wonder what is the ideal pressure that they should be using with the circle grip. An easy answer to this is to use enough force to move blood across the shaft, but nothing that feels uncomfortable or causes pain.

When you move the circle grip across the shaft and stop right at the glans, you have successfully performed a single repetition. When you reach this point, you can then use your other hand to perform the exact same motion.

This way, you can really perform several repetitions in a short amount of time.

If possible, try to shave the genital area that comes in contact with your hands when doing the jelqing motions. Although it is possible to perform jelqing with pubic hair, it can sometimes make things more difficult, especially if you're not using enough lubricant.

It is very important that you familiarize yourself with the jelqing motion, as it is one of the most important exercises in male enhancement. You will probably find yourself coming back to this exercise several times until you reach your desired size goals. Jelqing can also be done if you simply want the male sex benefits of improved erections and blood flow.

Manual stretching

If jelqing is the king of male enhancement exercises, then the manual stretch is arguably the queen or the heir to the throne. It is an extremely basic exercise, and probably the first male enhancement exercise to be performed by a human being due to how easy it is to do. Jelqing is a bit more complex in comparison, as it requires more prep work and steps.

Jelqing helps increase the overall size of the penis, although it is probably a bit biased towards thickness. Stretching, on the other hand, is used mainly for length gains. The length gains you can get from manual stretching can be very impressive. While it is possible to improve thickness slightly with manual stretching, keep in mind that his exercise should be used mostly for length.

Manual stretches are also typically performed first in several male enhancement routines, mainly because they help warm-up the ligaments and penis tissue so that you can have an easier time performing more complex exercises later.

You might have performed a basic stretch several times during your life already, without knowing that a similar motion is used to increase length; however, it is highly unlikely that you used enough intensity or time to trigger growth.

To perform a stretch, grab the penis from the glans and then stretch it as much as you can without getting to the point where you feel pain. The stretches are usually performed at several angles to trigger growth as much as possible. It is also essential to perform each stretch for several seconds.

It is crucial to remember that you shouldn't be feeling pain when performing this exercise. Because of how simple it is to perform, it is also easy to go overboard with it. The only thing you should be feeling is a minor tingly sensation across the shaft of the penis.

Pain is not a good indicator of progress in male enhancement. "The no pain, no gain" rule is used a lot in sports, but it doesn't apply here. Remember that the tissue of the penis is quite delicate, and pain is always a red flag that lets you know that you should back off either in intensity or frequency. You do this by using less force when performing the exercise and by doing fewer repetitions. In some cases, it might be necessary to include more rest days, where you don't do any male enhancement exercises at all.

Helicopter shake

Helicopter shakes are great for warming up and increasing blood flow in the penis. Although they don't stimulate growth directly, they are one of the best exercises that you can have in your toolkit. For some people, it can be challenging to perform stretches or jelqs without really loosening up things by doing helicopter shakes.

It is a good idea to include helicopter shakes at the start of your male enhancement routines. You shouldn't be doing jelqs or stretches without proper warmup first.

If you have ever twirled a set of keys before, then keep in mind that same movement when performing helicopter shakes. You start by grabbing the penis right at the base, as close as the pubic bone as possible. I recommend using a circle grip similar to the one you used when jelqing.

You then twirl your penis in a circle by using your wrist, just like you do when spinning your car or house keys. You can rotate your penis both clockwise and counterclockwise. It is recommended to go in both directions. Completing a circle means that you have successfully performed a repetition.

V-Jelqing

V-jelqs are one of the most versatile and practical exercises in male enhancement. Typically, most exercises have a significant bias towards either length or thickness, but V-jelqs tend to be helpful for both. If you are having trouble finding enough time to perform male enhancement exercises, then v-jelqs should be one of the exercises you should often be doing, as they are great at saving time.

The v-jelqing motion is very similar to what would happen if you mixed standard jelqs and manual stretching. It combines the best of both worlds. It might sound a complicated exercise that is not suitable for beginners, but in reality, the v-shaped jelq is often recommended to those that are starting, and thus you will see it in many newbie programs.

To perform a V-jelq you begin by cupping your hand in a V-shape. You create the V by joining the pinky with the ring finger and the index with the middle finger. Separate both pairs of fingers so that it seems as though you are performing the famous salute done in Star Trek. Curl up your hand a bit into a cup position and insert the penis in the V-shaped groove in your hand. If the underside of your penis is resting in your hand, you are on the right track. The penis should be firmly gripped by the V-groove, and you should also hold it very close to the pubic bone, just like when performing a standard jelq or helicopter shake.

After this, you then perform an upward pulling motion and stop right when you reach the glans.

It might sound like you are performing a very similar movement to standard jelqs, and that is true; however, a big difference between the two exercises is that in V jelqs, the penis is also pulled towards several angles, just like you do when performing manual stretches. When you reach the glans with the cupping hand, you have successfully completed a repetition, and you then make the same motion with the other hand. Just as with jelqs, using a lubricant helps make things smoother.

V-shaped jelqs should be mainly done with a level two erection (50%) or even less. It's very difficult and dangerous to stretch and pull the penis when there is too much blood in the shaft.

Kegels

You've probably heard about Kegels before. They aren't exclusive for men too: they are often recommended to women for several reasons. Another name for Kegels is pelvic floor exercises. Doctors usually recommend them to people that have urinary incontinence or pelvic floor issues.

When you perform Kegels, you're helping strengthen the pelvic floor muscles, which help support several organs such as the bladder, the uterus, and the rectum.

Although Kegels won't be adding any size to your penis, they are one of the best complementary exercises that you can add to a male enhancement routine.

Men that perform Kegel exercises regularly report several benefits such as better ejaculation control (they are an excellent tool for men that suffer from premature ejaculation), better ejaculation strength, improved ejaculation strength, and enhanced intensity of orgasms.

Adding Kegels to a routine is extremely simple and helps promote the growth and repair of the penis tissue. Because of the increased blood flow that Kegels improve in the genital area, the penis recovers much faster from the micro-tears caused by male enhancement exercises. Kegels will help you avoid setbacks as they are handy to prevent overtraining.

A great thing about Kegels is that they are effortless to perform. You can do them while sitting, which means that you can do them while working or driving. You can perform Kegels any time that you are doing other activities, which makes them very time efficient.

Kegels can be quite tricky to perform at first because a lot of people don't know how to locate the pubococcygeus. If you've ever stopped the flow of urine, then that's the same muscle that you need to contract to perform a repetition. An easy way to locate the pubococcygeus is to sit on a solid surface such as a chair and then attempt to recruit the same muscle you used to stop the flow of urine. Sitting down on a solid surface quickly helps develop a reliable mind to muscle connection.

When you contract the muscle, you have successfully performed one repetition. You can do Kegel repetitions in quick succession, but you may choose to hold the contractions for several seconds. Beginners might find it hard to contract the muscle for longer than one second though. More intermediate and advanced users can easily contract the PC muscles for several seconds.

Horse squeezes

Horse squeezes are very popular with advanced users. Definitively not an exercise for beginners, as there are other easier to perform exercises that will give similar results. However, men that want to continue to gain more size, after a certain point may realize that they need to use specific exercises to trigger more growth beyond the newbie and intermediate phase.

Horse squeezes have been used successfully by some men to break through plateaus. They mainly help with girth gains, but they can also be useful for gaining length. A proper warm-up is essential when performing this exercise

To perform a horse squeeze correctly, it is necessary to use an erection level of 3 or 4.

You start by using either of your hands to make the same circle grip we've used before for jelqing and then grip the base of the penis, as close to the pubic bone as you can. Squeeze the base of the penis in such a way that the blood doesn't escape. You can loosen the grip a bit and contract the PC muscle (the same one used to perform a Kegel rep) until your erection gets to the point you want it to be. The other hand should be used to perform another circle grip, one that is smaller in size. This smaller circle grip should be placed at the glans and should be moved through the shaft until it touches the base grip.

This movement has to be done quite slow to make it useful. A single repetition should last anywhere from fifteen to thirty seconds. When making this motion, you will displace blood inside the penis glans and create a lateral expansion of the tunica. There is a lot of internal pressure involved with this exercise, so it's best done after other milder exercises such as jelqs and stretches.

CHAPTER 4: MALE ENHANCEMENT ROUTINE FOR BEGINNERS

If you wish to gain size as quickly as possible, then it is essential to minimize setbacks as much as you can. A lot of men that discover male enhancement become very enthusiastic at the fact that they can modify their penis size permanently by doing exercises or using devices. Because of this, they think that by doing as much they can, they will get results quickly. This is not only inaccurate but can be quite dangerous. Male enhancement exercises are very safe when performed correctly, but when done excessively and with little care, it is possible to damage the penis tissue. Because of this, the best way to reach your size goals without setbacks is by following a routine that has the right exercises and frequency for your current stage.

The beginner program in this chapter includes exercises that the vast majority of untrained men will benefit from. The frequency and exercises are optimal for the average unconditioned penis.

As a bare minimum, you should try to stick with the beginner program for at least four months. It is normal for some men not to see any significant growth after four months. However, if you continue to see growth after the four-month mark, then feel free to stick with the program. It is when you stop seeing gains when it makes the most sense to switch to the intermediate routine.

You can also go back to the beginner routine at any point in your life when you would like to receive a boost in penis health. The exercises included help with erections and stamina too.

For some men, all they need to reach their size goals is to stick with the beginner's program for at least 4-6 months.

If you feel like you've reached a point where you are happy with your current size, then it is not necessary at all to do the intermediate program. If you wish to continue gaining in size, then you should move to the next level.

How often to train

There is not a set rule on how often to train for male enhancement. Generally speaking, most men will do fine when training five consecutive days and then resting for two days. Some men can tolerate more and are able to train for six straight days and rest for one. Men that can't tolerate much would do better if they do the exercises two days in a row and then rest for one. It is up to you to check what type of frequency would work best.

If you have a hectic life and find it very hard to take some time in your schedule to perform the routines, then even doing the program for two days per week will give results. Remember that the more often you perform the exercises while avoiding overtraining will provide you with the best and quickest results possible.

How to warm-up

Not all male enhancement programs include a warm-up phase, but this can be a big mistake, especially in beginner programs, since newbies aren't used to the kind of stress that male enhancement exercises place on the penis. A lot of times, setbacks can be completely avoided with a warm-up. 5-10 minutes of warm-up is recommended. Even if you can only manage the bare minimum of 5 minutes, that is much better than not doing any at all.

The ideal way to warm up is to soak a piece of cloth in mildly hot water.

Check first that the water is just slightly warm and not very hot.

You then place the towel and rub it through your whole genital and pubic area. The wet cloth should reach the penis shaft, glans, base, testicles and pubic region.

After applying the hot water for a while, the moistened areas should start to feel quite warm from the inside. Feeling this tells you that you are prepared to move on to the exercises.

Exercise 1. Two sets of helicopter shakes

-Perform 80 repetitions of helicopter shakes clockwise.

-Perform 80 repetitions of helicopter shakes counter-clockwise.

As you can see, we are slowly moving up the ladder of intensity. The first exercise we do is the helicopter shake, which is also a great exercise to promote blood flow and prepare things for more strenuous exercises.

Exercise 2. Manual stretches.

You will then perform manual stretches using different angles. The stretches are done for a set amount of time, so its best to use a timer instead of trying to guess how much time has gone by.

Imagine that the penis is located right in the middle of an imaginary clock. As reference, if you pull your penis straight up, that's a 12 o'clock position. If you pull straight down, then that would be at a 6 o´clock position.

First set of stretches

Pull the penis to a 6 o´clock position for 20 seconds.

Pull the penis to a 12 o´clock position for 20 seconds.

Pull the penis to a 3 o´clock position for 20 seconds.

Pull the penis to a 9 o´clock position for 20 seconds.

After hitting those four different angles, grab and stretch the penis starting from the 12 o´clock position and slowly make a full circle with it, clockwise. Maintain the same amount of tension while you perform the circle and keep it fully stretched at all times. The circle should last 50-60 seconds.

Second set of stretches

During the second set, you will be hitting a different set of angles. It's crucial to hit many different angles and not just two or three.

Pull the penis to a 1 o´clock position for 20 seconds.

Pull the penis to a 2 o´clock position for 20 seconds.

Pull the penis to a 11 o´clock position for 20 seconds.

Pull the penis to a 10 o´clock position for 20 seconds.

Pull the penis to a 4 o´clock position for 20 seconds.

Pull the penis to a 5 o´clock position for 20 seconds.

Pull the penis to an 8 o´clock position for 20 seconds.

Pull the penis to a 7 o´clock position for 20 seconds.

To finish the second set of stretches, grab the penis at the 12 o´clock position and make another circle similar to the first one, but this time, using a counter-clockwise direction. This circle should also be performed slowly, trying to make it last anywhere from 50-60 seconds.

Exercise 3. Jelqing

Jelqing tends to stress the penis tissue more than manual stretches, which is why it is best to perform them after there has been some decent amount of warm-up done beforehand.

As mentioned before, try to use lubricant and shave the pubic region if possible so that you can perform the movement more fluidly. Never go past a level 3 erection. Try to keep your erection between levels 1-3 only.

First set of jelqs.

The first set of jelqs will consist of performing rapid repetitions.

Perform 50 repetitions one after another by using both hands. Repetitions should last no more than one second.

Second set of jelqs

Now it's time to do slow repetitions.

Perform 50 repetitions, one after another, but this time, each motion should last around 3-4 seconds.

After performing both sets of jelqs, you can either warm down, by doing the same process with the wet towel you did when warming up, (however, you can do it for a shorter amount of time this time. 3-4 minutes is enough) or do V-jelqs. If you are a complete beginner, we recommend going straight to the warm down phase. After performing the exercises for 1-2 months, feel free to add in the V-Jelqs.

Exercise 4. V Jelqs.

Never go beyond a level 2 erection when performing V Jelqs.

Do 20 repetitions of V Jelqs by pulling the penis towards a 12 o´clock angle.

Do 20 repetitions of V Jelqs by pulling the penis towards a 6 o´clock angle.

Do 20 repetitions of V Jelqs by pulling the penis towards a 3 o´clock angle.

Do 20 repetitions of V Jelqs by pulling the penis towards a 9 o´clock angle.

Each repetition can last anywhere from one to three seconds.

How to train smart and avoid setbacks

Once you perform the routine several times, you can assess how your body is responding to it by checking for positive or negative signs of progress. For permanent gains, the process is usually as follows:

1.   You will first start noticing an improvement in erection quality.

2.   After your erection quality improves for a few days, you should begin to see an increase in size. Veins might become more prominent, too, at this point. All of this is positive. They're good signs that let you know that what you've been doing has been good.

3.   If you continue creating micro-tears in the penis tissue with enough recovery, you'll eventually arrive at a permanent increase in size. Even if you stopped doing the exercises, you should be able to retain most of the size you've gained.

On the other hand, if you start to notice that your penis isn't as sensitive as before, or if there is a decrease in erection quality, that is a very good indicator that you're probably training too much. If you start to notice this, it is important to take at least 3-4 days off to allow your body to heal before you continue with the routines.

If you aren't noticing a positive or negative sign, then that means that you are not stimulating the penis tissue enough. You can reduce your rest days or slightly increase the intensity of the exercises that you've been doing.

For a lot of men, male enhancement will be a very smooth ride. Some men are fortunate and have penises that can withstand lots of exercise. These men very rarely get overtrained, If at all. Other men might find it trickier to get the balance of rest and exercise right. For these men, the only way to move forward is through constant trial and error. By experimenting with the intensity and frequency they will eventually find something that lets them progress without any setbacks. Tolerance to exercise is extremely individual and can vary a lot among men.

CHAPTER 5: MALE ENHANCEMENT ROUTINE FOR INTERMEDIATE USERS

As mentioned in the previous chapter, the beginner program will decrease in effectiveness after using it consistently for several months. If it has been a few weeks since you've seen any size increases, then it's a good time to move on to the intermediate program.

Just as your muscles would adapt to an exercise routine and you'd then need to find something different to continue stimulating them, the penis will adjust to similar levels of force and tension; this means that the tissue won't need to adapt and thus grow.

The intermediate program shares a few similarities with the beginner program, but it has racked up the intensity a little.

How to warm-up

Being past the beginner stage doesn't mean that you can skip the warm-up. Good warm-up will always be necessary to minimize the possibility of injuries and overtraining. The same 5-10 minutes of warm-up with the wet towel that you did in the beginner's program will be useful here.

After the warm-up, doing the two sets of helicopter shakes, 60 reps each (clockwise and counter-clockwise) is optional. However, if you find yourself overtraining at some point while doing the intermediate program, then it might be a good idea to include the helicopter shakes and maybe even increase your current warm up time.

Exercise 1. Manual stretches.

First set of stretches.

Pull the penis to a 6 o'clock position for 30 seconds.

Pull the penis to a 12 o'clock position for 30 seconds.

Pull the penis to a 3 o'clock position for 30 seconds.

Pull the penis to a 9 o'clock position for 30 seconds.

After hitting those four different angles, grab and stretch the penis starting from the 12 o'clock position and slowly make a full circle with it, clockwise. Maintain the same amount of tension while you perform the circle and keep it fully stretched at all times.

The circle should last 50-60 seconds. This remains unchanged from the beginner program.

Second set of stretches

It is now time to hit new angles that will help promote growth. You need to do these by pulling the penis from under your legs, behind your glutes (as if the penis was a tail).

From the "tail" position, pull the penis to the right for 30 seconds.

From the "tail" position, pull the penis to the left for 30 seconds.

From the "tail" position, pull the penis down for 30 seconds.

From the "tail" position, pull the penis right at the center for 30 seconds.

After hitting these four different angles, it's time to do another full circle, but this time do it from the "tail" position. It should also last 50-60 seconds.

Exercise 2. Jelqing

The next exercise is jelqs. You can now try to perform them at a higher erection level. If you were using a level 1 or 2, you could try doing them with a level 3. However, it is still important not to go past a level 3.

First set of jelqs.

The first set of jelqs will consist of performing rapid repetitions.

Perform 100 repetitions one after another by using both hands. Repetitions should last no more than one second.

Second set of jelqs

Now it's time to do slow repetitions.

Perform 100 repetitions, one after another, but this time, each motion should last around 3-4 seconds.

Exercise 3. V Jelqing

There are no changes with the erection level that you use to perform V Jelqs.

Never go past a level 2 erection when performing them, as they will be tough.

Do 30 repetitions of V Jelqs by pulling the penis towards a 12 o´clock angle.

Do 30 repetitions of V Jelqs by pulling the penis towards a 6 o´clock angle.

Do 30 repetitions of V Jelqs by pulling the penis towards a 3 o´clock angle.

Do 30 repetitions of V Jelqs by pulling the penis towards a 9 o´clock angle.

Each repetition can last anywhere from one to three seconds.

Finish the intermediate program by warming down with the wet towel. Anywhere from 3-5 minutes is good enough.

CHAPTER 6: Male enhancement
ROUTINE FOR ADVANCED USERS

Just like with the beginner's program, there will be a certain point where you will stop seeing any progress after you've followed the intermediate plan for a while. The body is continuously adapting to the stress we throw at it, which eventually makes some of the methods we've used to increase in size so far ineffective.

If you find that you would like to continue making gains after you've stopped growing from the intermediate program, then here is an advanced program that will help trigger new growth. This program includes horse squeezes, an exercise that is best reserved for advanced users only, as it can easily cause overtraining if the penis tissue isn't used to the levels of stress.

Warm-up

The warm-up remains unchanged. Never forget to include at least 5 minutes of warm-up with the wet towel.

Exercise 1. Manual stretches.

First set of stretches.

Pull the penis to a 6 o´clock position for 43 seconds.

Pull the penis to a 12 o´clock position for 43 seconds.

Pull the penis to a 3 o´clock position for 43 seconds.

Pull the penis to a 9 o´clock position for 43 seconds.

After hitting those four different angles, grab and stretch the penis starting from the 12 o´clock position and slowly make a full circle with it, clockwise. Maintain the same amount of tension while you perform the circle and keep it fully stretched at all times. The circle should last 50-60 seconds.

Second set of stretches

From the "lion's tail" position, pull the penis to the right for 43 seconds.

From the "lion's tail" position, pull the penis to the left for 43 seconds.

From the "lion's tail" position, pull the penis down for 43 seconds.

From the "lion's tail" position, pull the penis right at the center for 43 seconds.

After hitting these four different angles, it's time to do another full circle, but this time do it from the "lion's tail" position. It should also last 50-60 seconds.

Exercise 2. Jelqing

The next exercise is jelqs. Continue performing them at a higher level than what you used in the beginner's program, but never go past level 3.

First set of jelqs.

The first set of jelqs will consist of performing rapid repetitions.

Perform 150 repetitions one after another by using both hands. Repetitions should last no more than one second.

Second set of jelqs

Now it's time to do slow repetitions.

Perform 150 repetitions, one after another, but this time, each motion should last around 3-4 seconds.

Exercise 3. The horse squeeze.

You need to perform a single horse squeeze only, as it is quite an intense exercise. Aim for 5-10 seconds of duration in total. You can add a second to every new session. Once you reach 40 seconds, don't add any more.

Finish the advanced program by performing a cooldown. Try to extend the cool-down period to at least 5 minutes, as the last exercise was quite intense.

CHAPTER 7: How to keep your gains

If you've gone through some of the programs included in this guide, you might be asking yourself what would happen if you completely stopped doing the exercises. If you've gone to the gym and lifted weights, you might have noticed that if you stop stimulating your muscles, you will eventually revert to your previous size. In some cases, you will be able to keep some of your muscle gains, but there will be an inevitable decrease.

The great news about exercising the penis is that this doesn't happen, to an extent. A good rule of thumb is to shoot for a little more when setting your size goals. For instance, if you wanted to increase the length of your penis 1.5 inches, then shoot for 2 inches.

After doing male enhancement and stopping cold turkey, some men report a loss of .5 inches.

If you reach your size goals (including the extra .5 inch) during the beginner program or the intermediate program, then it's not necessary to move to the next program. There is no harm in doing the program indefinitively, as you will get benefits such as improved erection quality, ejaculation control, etc. At some point in your life, you might want to improve in those areas, so you may go back to a male enhancement routine for some time if you need the boost. When done safely, male enhancement routines can be a great addition to your sex life.

CHAPTER 8: COMMON QUESTIONS ABOUT MALE ENHANCEMENT

You might have some questions about male enhancement, so I'll try to cover the most common ones here. Please keep in mind that some of these might have already been covered in previous chapters, but because of their importance should be mentioned again.

1.   What is a good size to shoot for?

A: Nobody can tell you what is the best size that you should set for yourself as a goal. Realistically speaking, most men can easily gain anywhere from 2-3 inches by following male enhancement exercise routines. Some might be able to gain even more size, but 2-3 inches is very realistic.

For a lot of men, even a single inch can make an enormous difference in their lives.

Some men get very ambitious and want to go for the biggest penis they can have. It is essential to realize that having a huge penis isn't always better. A lot of sex partners won't be able to feel very comfortable with large penises, as they can cause pain during intercourse.

2.   How is it possible for the penis to increase in size permanently by doing male enhancement exercises?

A: Whenever you expose the tissue of your penis to force, you'll create micro-tears from the damage. Your body knows about this and realizes that it is important to repair those micro tears or "something bad might happen." Your body knows that it is crucial to adapt to stress. With enough exercise and recovery days, your body will repair the microtears, which makes way for growth.

3.   I've skipped the warm-up phase for a while, and I've been ok. Should I continue like this?

A: Some men will be able to get away with skipping the warm-up and apparently won't have setbacks.

However, in most cases, it is just a matter of time until overtraining catches up with them. Because of this, make it a priority to warm-up appropriately before starting with the exercises.

4.   I don't want to cause any unwanted side effects by doing male enhancement exercises. Can I cause any permanent damage?

A: When done correctly, male enhancement exercises are healthy and safe. Of course, you should be consulting with your physician before beginning any male enhancement routine. Every man's body is different and will have a different response to the exercises, but it is crucial to remember that it is never ok to experience pain.

The penis is a delicate organ, so it is essential to pay attention to anything that our body is telling us. If you ever feel any pain or discomfort, then it is vital to immediately back off. Include more rest days, reduce the intensity/force that you use while doing the exercises, or both.

All of the following are warning signs that something is wrong and you should back off from exercising:

-Loss of erection quality.

-Any pain in the penis or testicles.

-Vein thrombosis.

-Loss of libido.

-In severe cases, short term erectile dysfunction.

5.   How can I know if I'm using enough force to stimulate growth when doing manual stretches?

A: Manual stretches can be tricky for inexperienced users because if you use little force, no growth will be triggered, and if you use too much force, you can easily cause pain and discomfort. The most common sensation that men report when doing manual stretches the right way is that of a slight sense of itchiness or tingling on the penis shaft. Be careful: itching or tingling isn't the same as pain. If you ever feel pain, then you should be using considerably less force.

6.   I don't like following exercise routines, can't I pick and choose some exercises and do them whenever I want to?

A: You don't need a male enhancement routine to make progress.

However, I highly recommended you to follow the programs because they are probably the easiest and quickest way to reach your size goals. If you pick and choose some exercises and do them whenever you feel like, then it is much more likely to either overtrain yourself or to not be triggering enough growth.

The three programs included in this guide help you get to your goals while avoiding as many bumps in the road as possible.

7.   Can I use a male enhancement device while I'm following a program?

A: It is not recommended to use a device while following the male enhancement routines, because they weren't designed with the use of a device in mind. Each device stresses the penis in a certain way, so it would be a challenging task to develop a program that is 100% compatible with devices.

It is possible to add a device, but then it would be even more important to pay attention to what your body is telling you, as you would be adding additional stress to the penis tissue.

8.   Are there any supplements that could help improve the gains made from the exercise routines?

A: It is not necessary to take any supplements to make good gains when following the routines, as there is no evidence yet of supplements that have shown to be useful for this purpose. You might want to take a few supplements that have been found to promote male sex health, such as Omega 3's, Ginseng, and Zinc. But always consult with a physician before starting to take any of these.

CHAPTER 9: HOW TO FIX PREMATURE EJACULATION

One of the most frustrating things that can happen to a man during sexual intercourse is premature ejaculation. If you're currently having problems with this, your case is far from unique: it is estimated that premature ejaculation affects around 20% of men at some point during their lives. In some cases the issue is not big enough to warrant serious attention, but in certain instances it can have devastating effects.

Premature ejaculation is usually attributed to teenagers and young adults, but it can happen at pretty much any stage of a man's life. In severe cases, it might cause severe self-esteem and psychological issues and can even negatively affect relationships.

Let's define what premature ejaculation is and why it happens. Premature ejaculation occurs when a man has an uncontrolled orgasm before his partner can achieve orgasm or enjoy sex. If this happens on multiple occasions, there is definitively a premature ejaculation issue.

In most cultures, if a man isn't able to last at least 4-7 minutes regularly during penetration, then most physicians would agree that he is having problems controlling his ejaculation.

The severity of premature ejaculation varies a lot. In some extreme cases, a man achieves an uncontrolled orgasm even before penetration starts. The physical touch from his partner or visual stimulation is enough for him to achieve an orgasm.

For a lot of men, premature ejaculation can cause them to suffer from extreme anxiety issues during sexual intercourse.

In some instances, anxiety might occur even before and after sex or sexual activity. Unfortunately, the concern only aggravates the problem, as one of the critical elements of good ejaculation control is relaxation.

There are two types of premature ejaculation: lifelong premature ejaculation and secondary premature ejaculation, also known as acquired premature ejaculation.

It is not always easy treating premature ejaculation because it is often linked to other issues. For instance, bad habits are a common cause. A classic example of this is boys and teenagers that tend to masturbate quickly to get to orgasm as soon as possible.

This habit, unfortunately, hinders them later on when they have sexual intimacy, as their bodies have been trained through countless repetitions to achieve orgasm as quickly as possible. These patterns can often be solved by simply addressing the root issues, in this case, slowing down the pace at which they masturbate. If these habits aren't fixed, then the problem might carry over to the man's life as an adult.

Secondary premature ejaculation usually occurs during adulthood. The cause is often but is not limited to, psychological issues. A typical pattern for secondary premature ejaculation happens when a man has an unpleasant experience during his first sexual contact.

Some health conditions can also have a significant impact on ejaculation control. Blood pressure, for instance and hormonal disbalances are known for affecting a man's ejaculation control.

In several cases, premature ejaculation can get better on its own. It is typical for a teenager or a young man that has premature ejaculation to overcome the problem without putting much thought into it. Sometimes, simply getting used to new sensations and stimulus is enough to improve ejaculation control.

As simple as it may sound, more practice can be the best antidote for poor ejaculation control. This is why premature ejaculation is an issue that is often present in younger, more inexperienced men.

Jelqing and ejaculation control

Male enhancement exercises can work wonders to improve one's ejaculation control. Jelqing and Kegels can be great tools for this purpose. Out of all the exercises available, Kegels are probably the ones that will have the most impact on your ability to control your orgasm.

Having weak pelvic floor muscles means that your orgasms will be weaker, and your ejaculation control will be reduced. Kegels strengthen the pelvic floor muscles and can improve contractions during orgasm. Doing at least three sets of 10 repetitions of Kegels (trying to hold each contraction for at least three seconds) works great in lots of cases.

Lifestyle changes

Positive lifestyle changes can also give good results. For example, reducing alcohol or tobacco intake and eating a healthier diet can help alleviate the anxiety that happens before, during, or after sexual intercourse, which is often one of the main contributors to the problem.

Being overly stressed is also a common cause of secondary premature ejaculation.

Certain short term fixes can be lifesavers.

Sometimes, wearing a thicker condom can help decrease the sensitivity of the penis, assisting men in delaying their ejaculation. Some condoms even have a substance inside that helps numb the penis slightly. These substances are also sold separately. Lidocaine is often used as a safe numbing agent for this purpose. The downside to using a numbing agent is that overall pleasure will be slightly decreased. Sometimes, even erection quality may also suffer.

The first thing to try for men that are suffering from premature ejaculation and have already done lifestyle changes is to try some of the following options:

Edging

Edging, or the stop-start technique is one of the easiest ways to practice ejaculation control, even without a partner. You can also do it with a partner, but at first, I suggest trying it by yourself.

Partners can get frustrated if you interrupt penetration often, which is done regularly in this exercise.

To practice the stop-start technique, you start by masturbating normally, but completely stop as you begin to feel that you are about to ejaculate. Imagine that there is a scale of 1-10, with one being almost not aroused at all, and ten meaning reaching ejaculation.

Practicing edging helps you become more conscious of where your current level of stimulation is.

A lot of times, premature ejaculation happens when men have very little awareness of their stimulation level. Before they know it, they reach the point of no return and ejaculate before they intended.

As you masturbate, you want to avoid going past levels 7 or 8 of stimulation. Once you go beyond a 7 or an 8 it can be tough to stop.

If you feel like you are reaching the point of no return, completely stop stimulating your penis and relax by taking several deep breaths. Make sure that your arousal level goes back to at least a 5 before continuing. If you only go back to a 6 or a 7, you will very quickly approach the point of no return again. It is better to take a pause and relax before continuing. This might take a few seconds, a minute or more in some cases.

After doing this exercise on multiple occasions, you will have developed an increased awareness of your levels of stimulation, helping you know exactly where you are the next time you are having sexual intercourse. Being aware that you are reaching a level 6 or 7 can help you realize that it might be a good idea to switch positions, reduce the speed of the penetration, or take a few deep breaths to help you relax.

Some partners might feel frustrated that you are interrupting penetration so often, so it is a good idea to mix in manual or oral stimulation while you get back to a "safer" level of arousal; by using your mouth or fingers to please your partner, you will take away a lot of the frustration of doing the stop-start technique during intercourse.

Male sex toys

There are male sex toys available that simulate the sensations of the vagina. They can be a powerful tool when combined with edging, as you will be able to not only make masturbation sessions more fun but also make them feel closer to what real sex feels. Manual stimulation often doesn't come close to the same level of stimulation that a vagina gives.

The squeeze technique

This is best used as a "last resort" option. If you notice that you are nearing ejaculation, then you can try squeezing your penis by pressing the area between the shaft and glans. When done correctly, this helps decrease the level of stimulation in the penis and helps go back to a level where you have better ejaculation control.

The squeeze technique doesn't do much if you are at a level 9 or 10. At that point, there is little you can do to go back to a more controlled state.

Also, it is best if you only do it a maximum of three times per session, as it can affect your erection quality.

Having more sex

This might sound like obvious advice, but it can be one of the main reasons why adult men tend to have better ejaculation control than teenagers. Getting used to the stimulus and sensations that happen during sex helps improve your ejaculation control and awareness. By having sex more often, you will also decrease performance anxiety, which is often one of the causes of premature ejaculation.

Ejaculating before sexual intercourse

This is one of the oldest pieces of advice, but don't discount it for that. It can still be beneficial. It is not rocket science: not ejaculating for several days heightens the sensitivity of the penis. If you masturbate a few hours before sexual intercourse, your penis will be much less sensitive.

However, you must know where your boundaries lie. If you know that you won't be able to have another erection in the next hour or two, then space the masturbation session further apart from sexual intercourse. If there is something worse than premature ejaculation, it could be not being able to achieve an erection at all!

Deep breathing

Deep breathing can also be used outside of the edging technique during intercourse.

A lot of men with excellent ejaculation control can hold off their orgasm thanks to their ability to remain relaxed. The pelvic floor muscles can quickly become tense if you're not relaxed, and before you know it, you've reached the point of no return.

If you remind yourself to take deep breaths for as much as you can during intercourse, then it is almost inevitable that you will feel more relaxed. After all, to relax our bodies, it all starts with our breathing.

To make sure you are taking deep breaths, inhale through your nose and exhale through your mouth, making sure that each breath lasts at least four seconds. By breathing deeply, you'll improve blood oxygenation, which then makes your brain release calming endorphins. Endorphins, also known as our "feel-good" hormones, help us feel happier and more relaxed.

Improving communication with your partner

Performance anxiety is often a cause of premature ejaculation. When a man feels pressured to perform during intercourse, he won't be able to relax, and before he knows it, reaches the point of no return.

In some cases, it can be very beneficial to have an honest conversation with your partner if you're feeling any pressure during sex.

Some cases might be more complex, and only a therapist might be able to solve them. For instance, some men have self-image issues that are very deeply rooted or a history of problems that might be contributing to the lack of relaxation during sex. Sometimes, only a professional can uncover the problems that are causing damage.

CHAPTER 10: HOW TO IMPROVE OR REVERSE ERECTILE DYSFUNCTION

It might surprise some to hear that the number one male sexual health problem reported to doctors isn't premature ejaculation, but erectile dysfunction. Fortunately, erectile dysfunction can often be reversed.

ED happens when there is a considerable amount of difficulty in getting or maintaining an erection that is firm enough for proper sexual intercourse. It is not uncommon for men to experience slight problems with their erections from time to time, but when the issue is present consistently, it then becomes a significant obstacle to overcome.

Just as with premature ejaculation, stress, anxiety, and emotional or psychological reasons might play a role in some cases.

In other cases, there could be problems with restricted blood flow in the penis. Erectile dysfunction is considered by some doctors to be an early sign of a more severe health issue such as heart disease, atherosclerosis or diabetes.

Why do erections happen?

For something that is such a big part of men's life, most don't know what causes erections in their bodies.

Whenever a man becomes sexually aroused, the nerves release chemicals that very quickly increase blood flow inside the penis. This blood goes into the two sponge-like regions of erectile tissue, the corpus cavernosa, which contains most of the blood that goes to the penis during an erection. The spongy tissue then relaxes to trap blood and maintain the erection.

The purpose of all of this is to make the penis firm enough to have sexual intercourse.

After ejaculation is reached, certain nerves then make the penis contract enough so that blood is released from the corpus cavernosa back to a man's circulation. As a result of this, the erection diminishes.

If a man is not sexually aroused, it is normal for the penis to be completely flaccid. Several external and internal factors might affect flaccid penis size, such as one's mood and the weather.

Erectile dysfunction happens when a man has trouble keeping or maintaining an erection when regularly having intercourse. Both psychological and physiological factors can cause ED.

Some of the most common physiological factors are:

-Certain health conditions, such as high blood sugar or hypertension.

-Overconsumption of alcohol, smoking, and other drugs.

-Getting little to no exercise.

-Age. Specifically, over 50 years old.

-Being overweight or obese.

Some of the most common physiological factors are:

-Mood disorders, such as depression or high levels of stress and anxiety.

-Unresolved relationship issues.

-Sexual performance anxiety.

Is it possible to reverse Erectile dysfunction?

ED is more easily treated than other male sex issues such as premature ejaculation because it has been studied far more extensively. Even when ED will not budge with lifestyle changes and therapy, there is treatment available that will do wonders to improve the condition.

-Primary erectile dysfunction is a very rare condition, and it is when a man has never been able to produce an erection in his life.

-Secondary erectile dysfunction is far more commonplace. Men that were previously able to have normal erections but are no longer capable of having them have secondary ED.

It is much easier to treat secondary ED than primary. Often, secondary ED is only temporary. Primary ED is a more severe condition that requires medical intervention and hormonal therapy or surgery in some cases.

How to treat erectile dysfunction

There are several ways to approach secondary ED, and it all depends on the root cause.

For instance, if the cause is a lack of blood flow in the genital region, there are drugs available that can significantly improve circulation in the penis. These types of drugs are mainly prescribed to men that are over the age of 50 or to men that are severely overweight. Sometimes, they are even prescribed to younger patients that are having ED problems to help them improve their quality of life.

If clogged arteries are the main issue and you wish to reverse the root cause of the problem, then by simply losing some weight, eating a healthier diet and exercising more, you will make enormous improvements to your erection quality.

Sometimes, hormonal deficiencies such as low testosterone can cause ED. Whenever there is a male sex issue present, one of the first things that physicians recommend is to have the patient's testosterone levels checked.

Low testosterone can cause a variety of different problems such as low libido, poor erection quality, brain fog, lack of energy, depression, etc.

If you check your testosterone levels and they are low enough, then your doctor will probably recommend you to make specific lifestyle changes. If those aren't sufficient, then you might be candidate for testosterone replacement therapy.

Certain medications are known for wreaking havoc in a man's sex life. Often, these meds have side effects that reduce testosterone production or decrease erection quality. If you are currently on medications and are experiencing any of these side effects, it's a good idea to talk to your physician and ask him if there are other options available that have less of those side effects.

In some milder cases, doing male enhancement exercises will be extremely beneficial to improve erection quality. After all, as you now know, one of the first signs that you have been performing the exercises correctly is an improvement in erection quality. If you do things right, you should start noticing firmer and stronger erections. Kegels can also help to improve and retain blood flow inside the corpus cavernosa of the penis.

Anxiety as a common cause of ED

Perhaps the most common physiological cause of ED is anxiety. There is even a name for the negative thoughts about the ability to perform well in the bedroom: performance anxiety. When a man has severe doubts or fears about their ability to perform or please their partner (these doubts can be influenced by several factors such as penis size, body image, ejaculation control, etc.), performance anxiety can rear its ugly head and make things even more challenging.

Performance anxiety can cause erectile dysfunction, premature ejaculation, and even the inability to achieve an orgasm (also known as delayed ejaculation).

The best way to protect yourself from performance anxiety is to avoid falling into its cycle. Once you are trapped in the cycle, it can be very challenging to deal with it.

If you have an unpleasant sexual experience (like losing ejaculation control or not being able to please your partner), avoid dwelling on the event, as it will only make you feel like a failure in the bedroom. It is very normal for men to not perform well from time to time. If you fall into the trap of dwelling on your bedroom failure, you will probably start feeling anxious before the next time you have sex. This then can develop a vicious cycle that causes many male sex issues.

Instead of using your mental energy and focus on obsessing with the negative event that happened, redirect your attention on trying to identify what happened so that you can improve next time, even if it was just a little. For instance, if you suffered from premature ejaculation because you have been extremely stressed from work lately, then it would be best to find methods to relax such as meditation, exercise, or therapy so that your worry and stress doesn't affect you next time.

Another good advice is to shift your focus to your senses next time that you start feeling anxiety during sex. Focus on touch, sound and what you're seeing. Pay attention to what your hands are doing, and what your skin is feeling. Using scented candles can be a great way to help you relax. By being fully present on what you're doing, there will be little room for worrying thoughts to creep in your mind.

Improving communication and talking openly with your partner can be one of the best antidotes for performance anxiety available. Your partner might not even know that there is an ongoing issue that has been affecting you. By opening up and speaking about the situation, she might help you find solutions to help with the problem. In some cases, sex therapy or even counseling for couples can be great to help with the issue.

As mentioned, erectile dysfunction is usually reversible and temporary. The above suggestions might work for a lot of men, but in some cases, only a visit to a doctor that has experience dealing with male sex issues will help you find the root cause of the issue and offer the right treatment.

CHAPTER 11: How to improve or
REVERSE ERECTILE DYSFUNCTION

No guide on male enhancement would be complete without explaining methods that help increase ejaculation. After all, ejaculation is a big part of male sexuality, and a lot of men are curious about how to improve it.

There have been recent studies done that show that a lot of men aren't satisfied with the current volume of their ejaculations. Just as with penis size, a lot of men have been exposed to porn videos where they see male adult actors ejaculating massive amounts of semen. Ejaculating large volumes of semen is seen as a sign of masculinity in a lot of cultures.

For a man, after having sex there is probably no better sight than seeing their big load covering certain parts of their partner's bodies.

For men, ejaculating a big load isn't the norm. The typical amount of liquid that a male ejaculates varies between three to five ml or about a teaspoon. There are lots of different factors that affect the size of ejaculation, with genetics and age being two of the biggest ones. For instance, the peak amount of volume that men ejaculate is during the years of 30-36. After this, the amount tends to diminish slowly with each passing year. This has been attributed to the normal decrease in testosterone that happens with age.

If you are or have been interested at some point in increasing the size of your ejaculation, then you might have wondered if there are things you can do to enhance it. Just as with size, the male enhancement industry is full of frauds and scams that won't do anything except for slimming your wallet.

Lots of pills and supplements are being sold that promise to increase your load.

Proven ways to increase your loads

Although it may sound like obvious advice, probably the easiest thing you can do to increase the volume of your loads as quickly as possible is to wait more time between ejaculations. Waiting for more than three days serves little purpose though, since the body fully replenishes semen reserves in three days. It is not always practical to wait three full days between ejaculations, but whenever you want to make a statement, keep this advice in mind.

To further enhance the size of your ejaculation, you must first understand what semen is made out of water, proteins, vitamins, amino acids, mineral. Contrary to popular belief, sperm only constitutes 1% of semen.

Being well hydrated

Because water is the most significant component of semen, if you are currently not drinking enough, the size of your loads will probably be much smaller than it can be. Simply by drinking more water and staying hydrated, the size of your loads will increase. Our body is made out of 60-70% water, so it's crucial to be well hydrated for all of our organs to function adequately. Make sure that you always have a bottle of water nearby, especially when you're not at home when it can be more difficult to access drinking water.

Weight and sperm count

Evidence shows that losing weight if you're currently overweight, will help increase the quantity of your semen. Men that are overweight or obese have less sperm count and a smaller volume of ejaculation than men with healthy body weight.

Some obese men have a practically nonexistent sperm count.

Helpful foods

Including more foods in your diet that are rich in antioxidants, zinc, chlorine, calcium, and vitamins A, C, B12 and D will also be beneficial to increase semen quality and quantity.

Because of their high antioxidant content, vegetables such as greens and berries are one of the best foods you can eat to increase ejaculation size.

There is one vegetable, though, that is famously known for promoting semen production: celery. Some well-known adult actors eat this vegetable often and recommend it to others that are also interested in increasing their load size.

It's not difficult to see why: Celery contains several of the vitamins and minerals that semen is made out of: vitamins A, C, potassium and folate.

Another crucial mineral is zinc, and it can be found in many different foods such as nut and seeds, legumes, eggs and meat. Men that are deficient in zinc often have low sperm counts and low libido. It's not hard to increase your weekly zinc intake; simply by eating more legumes, meats (depending on your type of diet) and eating a few handfuls of nuts should be enough. It's always a good idea to check with a blood test where your levels are.

Exercise and sleep

Although you already should be exercising at least 3-6 per week for overall health, if you want to produce as much semen as possible, you simply need to exercise regularly. The best types of exercise for this purpose are cardio and weight lifting.

Cardio exercise improves blood flow and weight lifting helps raise your testosterone levels.

Sleep is similar to exercise. Getting proper amounts of sleep is crucial to help our bodies recover and repair. If you're not currently getting 7-8 hours of sleep every night, your body won't be able to recover fully and semen production will decrease.

Supplements

There hasn't been enough research done on the impact of supplements in semen volume. However, a lot of men have reported success with certain supplements that are readily available in most vitamin or health shops. Sometimes, simply taking these supplements makes a big difference in semen size.

Here are some of the most commonly recommended supplements:

-Lecithin. Lecithin is made out of a combination of fatty acids, which may improve semen quality. It has been shown to improve the quality of semen in certain animals. The substance has been recognized by the U.S. food and drug administration to be safe for human consumption.

-L-arginine. This is usually taken to boos libido and stamina, but some men have reported that it also seems to promote stronger erections and improve ejaculation volume. It is not a typically recommended specifically for increasing semen size, but it can be used for this purpose. It is a very popular supplement with men of age 50 and beyond but it can also be taken by younger men that wish to boost their sexual performance.

-Ashwagandha. This is a very popular herb taken by people that tend to have problems with stress or anxiety. As stress (and thus cortisol levels) increase, testosterone production decreases.

It makes sense to take supplements such as ashwagandha to increase your testosterone levels if you're going through lots of daily stress.

-Butea Sueprba. A herb from Thailand that has been used to promote sexual health for a long time. A lot of people have reported that it can help with erectile dysfunction, low libido and increasing semen quantity.

Enhancing semen's taste

You've probably asked yourself what your semen tastes like at some point.

Some men are interested in enhancing the taste of their semen to help their partners enjoy oral sex more. A lot of men find pleasure in watching their partner swallow their load. However, lots of people have a difficult time swallowing semen because they usually can't stand the taste and find it very off-putting.

Semen taste can vary a lot, and it can go from something that tastes like battery acid to salty or even slightly sweet. Why is there such a wide range? Your body's ph levels, and lifestyle havbits are two of strongest factors that affect the taste of your semen. For instance, people that don't exercise regularly, eat lots of junk food and take drugs tend to have very bitter tasting semen.

Semen tends to have an alkaline ph level of 7 in order to protect the sperm once they're inside the vagina, which is an acidic environment.

Foods and substances that affect semen taste negatively

-Caffeine: drinking to much coffee or caffeinated drinks tends to result in bitter tasting semen.

-Excessive meat consumption: Eating too much meat tends to make semen taste more salty and bitter.

-Medicine: Certain meds make our body odor and bodily fluids smell worse. This includes sweat, urine and semen.

-Asparagus: You've probably noticed that your urine smells very strong after eating too much of this vegetable. It doesn't do any favors to the way your semen tastes either.

-Processed foods: Junk foods tends to have lots of chemicals that will affect the way your semen tastes.

Foods and substances that make semen taste better

-Water: As explained before, semen is mostly made out of water, so it's crucial to be properly hydrated. Drinking enough water will not only affect the volume of your semen but it's taste too.

-Celery: Similar to water, it has been reported by some men that celery increases both volume and taste of semen.

-Spices/herbs: Some spices such as sinammon and peppermint have been known for sweetening the taste of semen. Herbs such as parsley and wheatgrass have a similar effect.

-Fruits: Fruits can be amazing for making your semen taste better. You might have heard about pineapple, but blueberries, ccranberries, kiwis and plumbs also work.

The best way to ask to know how your semen tastes is to simply ask your partner. If they tell you that it doesn't taste pleasant, then it might be a good idea to try some of the suggestions made, and make adjustments so that it eventually tastes better. It's actually not that difficult to improve semen's taste, and the rewards are often worth it: oral sex sessions that are more satisfying to both you and your partner.

CONCLUSION

After reading this guide you are hopefully feeling excited about all of the different male enhancement options that you have at your disposal. How cool it is to realize that you can actually modify the size of your penis, improve your erections, stamina and even increase the volume of your semen and modify its tastes. All of these things are now largely under your control.

Living with anxiety about your penis size can be a living nightmare for lots of males. The same applies to not being able to pleasure your partner due to male sex problems such as erectile dysfunction or low libido. It's undeniable that men's self esteem is largely connected to their sexual performance and their penis size.

If you asked a lot of men what they would prefer if given the option: to become a millionaire or increase the size of their penis, a lot of them would choose to have a bigger penis. It's quite something to realize that you now have the tools to modify your penis to the size that you've always wished without having to use methods with horrible side effects.

Whatever your goal maybe, whether it is to simply increase your penis in size or to enhance your overall performance during sex, I hope that you now feel empowered and that you'll find an enhanced sense of confidence that will spill over to several areas of your time.

Thank you for reading this guide and good luck!

CPSIA information can be obtained
at www.ICGtesting.com
Printed in the USA
BVHW041458170220
572580BV00017B/500